Dedication

To my family,

May we always be as protected as we are blessed.

With all my love

Foreword

In emergencies, every second counts. The ability to respond swiftly and effectively can be the difference between life and death. This book is born out of a passion for empowering people with the knowledge and skills needed to save lives. Whether you're a concerned parent, a cautious traveler, or simply someone who wants to be prepared, this guide is designed for you.

With a focus on debunking common misconceptions and providing clear, actionable steps, this book aims to equip you with the essential tools to handle a variety of medical emergencies. Knowledge is power, and being prepared can make all the difference.

Thank you for taking the time to learn these critical skills. May this book be a valuable resource for you and those you care about.

Table of Contents

Introduction

In the blink of an eye, an ordinary day can turn into a life-or-death situation. Whether it's a car accident on a busy street, a sudden allergic reaction at a family picnic, or a severe laceration from a kitchen mishap, emergencies strike without warning. The real tragedy, however, often lies in the myths and misconceptions that surround these critical moments—misconceptions that can mean the difference between life and death.

Welcome to your indispensable guide to emergency first aid—a compact, no-nonsense booklet designed to equip you with the knowledge to save lives. This book strips away the fluff and filler, focusing solely on the essential facts and techniques you need to act swiftly and effectively in the face of medical emergencies.

Consider this: at any given moment, you could be the first responder. Whether you're at home, on the road, or out in public, the skills you'll learn here can prepare you to help someone in dire need or even save your own life. From handling a choking child to managing a heart attack, from properly applying a tourniquet to recognizing the signs of a stroke, this guide dispels dangerous myths and replaces them with clear, actionable steps.

Common misconceptions—like tilting your head back during a nosebleed or giving insulin during a diabetic ketoacidosis episode—are not just harmless errors. They are pervasive, often perpetuated by outdated advice and dramatized media portrayals. This book confronts these false beliefs head-on, providing you with the correct information to act decisively and confidently.

Designed for ease of use, this booklet is compact enough to fit in your purse, pocket, or glove compartment, ensuring that it's always within reach when you need it most. Its straightforward approach makes learning and recalling vital first aid techniques simple, even in the most stressful situations.

In these pages, you'll find:
- Clear instructions on what to do (and what not to do) in various emergencies.
- Insights into the myths that can lead to mistakes and how to avoid them.
- Practical, easy-to-remember mnemonics and steps for fast action.

Remember, emergencies don't wait for the perfect moment—they demand immediate action. Equip yourself with the knowledge and confidence to step in and make a difference. This book is your guide to being prepared, debunking the dangerous myths, and becoming a capable first responder whenever the need arises.

So, dive in, arm yourself with life-saving knowledge, and take the first step towards being a hero in an emergency. You never know when you might need it, but with this guide, you'll be ready when the time comes.

Chapter 1: Natural Emergencies

Natural emergencies can, and mostly will, strike without warning, turning life's ordinary moments into life-threatening situations. From heart attacks to strokes, these medical crises require immediate and informed responses to save lives.

This chapter delves into the most common natural emergencies, debunking myths and providing clear, actionable steps to ensure you can act swiftly and effectively.

Understanding these emergencies and knowing how to respond can make all the difference in critical moments, empowering you to be a lifeline when it's needed most.

Heart Attack

Misconception

Only older people have heart attacks, and they always involve severe chest pain.

When and How This Misconception Could Occur

This misconception is common in both laypersons and, occasionally, among medical professionals. It can occur in workplaces, public spaces, or homes when someone exhibits atypical symptoms that are not immediately recognized as a heart attack, especially in younger individuals.

Why This Thought is Popular

Heart attacks are often depicted as dramatic events involving clutching the chest and falling over, typically affecting older adults. This portrayal in media and general discussions reinforces the idea that severe chest pain is always present and that heart attacks primarily affect the elderly.

Reality

Heart attacks can occur at any age and may present with symptoms like shortness of breath, nausea, lightheadedness, or discomfort in other areas of the upper body. Chew an aspirin (if not allergic) and seek emergency medical help immediately.

When Heart Attacks Occur

Heart attacks can result from various factors, including

genetics, lifestyle, stress, and underlying health conditions. They can occur suddenly or develop over time, with symptoms ranging from mild to severe.

Why This Thought is Correct

Recognizing the diverse symptoms of a heart attack is critical for timely intervention. Not all heart attacks present with classic chest pain. Symptoms can include discomfort in the back, jaw, neck, or stomach, shortness of breath, nausea, and fatigue. Understanding this can lead to quicker response and better outcomes.

What You Can Do in That Situation

Steps to Handle a Suspected Heart Attack

1. **Recognize the Symptoms:** Be aware of both classic and atypical symptoms. These include chest pain or discomfort, pain in other areas of the upper body, shortness of breath, cold sweat, nausea, or lightheadedness.

2. **Call Emergency Services:** Immediately call 911 or your local emergency number. Do not attempt to drive the person to the hospital yourself.

3. **Provide Aspirin:** If the person is not allergic to aspirin, have them chew a standard adult aspirin (not swallow it whole) to help thin the blood.

4. **Keep the Person Calm:** Encourage the person to sit down and stay calm. Reassure them that help is on the way.

5. **Monitor Their Condition:** Stay with the person and monitor their symptoms. Be prepared to provide CPR if they lose consciousness and stop breathing.

Emotional Support and Communication

- **Stay Reassuring:** Keep a calm demeanor and provide continuous reassurance. Let the person know that medical help is on the way.
- **Communicate Clearly:** If the person is conscious, explain your actions and the steps you are taking to help them. This can help reduce their anxiety.
- **Offer Continuous Support:** Remain with the person, maintaining eye contact and providing comfort. Your presence and calm communication can significantly help in managing their stress and fear.

<u>Stroke</u>

Misconception

Wait to see if symptoms improve before seeking help.

When and How This Misconception Could Occur

This misconception can occur in homes, workplaces, or public spaces where someone exhibits mild or intermittent symptoms of a stroke. The reluctance to seek immediate help might stem from not recognizing the severity of the situation or assuming the symptoms will resolve on their own.

Why This Thought is Popular

Stroke symptoms can sometimes be mistaken for other less severe conditions like fatigue, dehydration, or stress. The idea to "wait and see" is often a result of underestimating the urgency and hoping that the problem will resolve without medical intervention.

Reality

If someone shows signs of a stroke (e.g., face drooping, arm weakness, speech difficulties), seek emergency medical help immediately. Time is critical in reducing the impact of a stroke.

When Strokes Occur

A stroke occurs when the blood supply to part of the brain is interrupted or reduced, depriving brain tissue of oxygen and nutrients. Symptoms include sudden numbness or weakness in the face, arm, or leg, especially on one side of the body; confusion; trouble speaking or understanding speech; difficulty seeing in one or both eyes; trouble walking; dizziness; and loss of balance or coordination.

Why This Thought is Correct

Immediate medical intervention can significantly reduce the damage caused by a stroke. The faster a person receives treatment, the better their chances of recovery and minimizing long-term effects. The "golden hour" is crucial for administering treatments that can dissolve clots or address bleeding in the brain.

What You Can Do in That Situation

Steps to Handle a Suspected Stroke

1. **Recognize the Symptoms:** Use the **FAST** acronym to identify stroke symptoms:

   - **Face:** Ask the person to smile. Does one side of the face droop?
   - **Arms:** Ask the person to raise both arms. Does one arm drift downward?
   - **Speech:** Ask the person to repeat a simple phrase. Is their speech slurred or strange?
   - **Time:** If you observe any of these signs, call 911 or emergency services immediately.

2. **Call Emergency Services:** Do not wait. Dial 911 or the local emergency number. Provide clear

information about the symptoms and the time they
started.

3. **Keep the Person Safe:** Ensure they are in a safe
    position, ideally lying down with their head slightly
    elevated.

4. **Stay with Them:** Keep the person calm and
    monitor their symptoms while waiting for
    emergency responders.

5. **Provide Relevant Information:** Inform the
    medical responders about the symptoms, any
    known medical conditions, and medications the
    person is taking.

Emotional Support and Communication

- **Stay Calm and Reassuring:** Speak in a calm and
  supportive manner. Reassure the person that help is
  on the way.
- **Encourage Compliance:** Encourage them to stay
  still and relaxed. Avoid giving food, drink, or
  medications.
- **Provide Continuous Support:** Stay with the
  person, offering comfort and reassurance until
  emergency medical personnel arrive.

Seizures

Misconception

During a seizure, you should restrain the person or put something in their mouth.

When and How This Misconception Could Occur

This misconception often arises in high-stress situations when bystanders panic and believe they need to "control" the person having the seizure to prevent self-injury. It's common in environments where first aid knowledge is limited or outdated. People might think that placing an object in the mouth prevents the person from swallowing their tongue, a widely held but incorrect belief.

Why This Thought is Popular

The idea of restraining someone or putting something in their mouth stems from a natural instinct to protect and prevent harm. It has been perpetuated through generations and popular media, where seizures are dramatized, and incorrect first aid actions are shown.

Reality

Do not restrain the person or put anything in their mouth. Clear the area of dangerous objects, cushion their head, and turn them on their side if possible. Stay with them until the seizure ends and they are fully alert.

When Seizures Occur

Seizures can occur due to a variety of reasons, including

epilepsy, high fever, head injury, low blood sugar, or other medical conditions. They often strike without warning and can be frightening for both the person experiencing the seizure and those around them.

Why This Thought is Correct

The correct response focuses on ensuring the safety of the person having the seizure without causing additional harm. Restraining them or putting something in their mouth can lead to injuries such as broken bones or aspiration. The person's body is reacting involuntarily, and the best course of action is to prevent further harm while allowing the seizure to run its course.

What You Can Do in That Situation

Steps to Help Someone Having a Seizure

1. **Stay Calm and Ensure Safety:** Clear the area of any objects that could cause injury, such as furniture or sharp items.

2. **Position the Person:** If possible, gently guide them to the ground and lay them on their side to keep their airway clear. Cushion their head with something soft like a jacket or pillow.

3. **Do Not Restrain:** Allow the seizure to proceed without trying to hold the person down. This reduces the risk of injury from the involuntary movements.

4. **Time the Seizure:** Note the duration of the seizure. If it lasts longer than 5 minutes, seek emergency medical help immediately.

5. **Stay With Them:** Remain by their side until the seizure ends and they regain full consciousness. Talk to them calmly and reassure them as they come around.

6. **Check for Injuries:** Once the seizure has stopped, check for any injuries they might have sustained during the episode. Offer support and comfort as they may be disoriented or tired.

Emotional Support and Communication

- **Stay Reassuring:** Speak calmly and offer comfort. Let them know they are safe and that you are there to help.
- **Explain What Happened:** Once they are alert, explain briefly what happened and reassure them that seizures are a medical condition and that help is available if needed.
- **Avoid Crowding:** Keep onlookers away to give the person privacy and prevent additional stress.

Severe Allergic Reaction (Anaphylaxis)

Misconception

Administering over-the-counter antihistamines can treat anaphylaxis.

When and How This Misconception Could Occur

This misconception might occur in situations where someone with a known allergy starts showing symptoms of a severe reaction. People might think that antihistamines, which are often used for mild allergic reactions, will be effective for anaphylaxis.

Why This Thought is Popular

Over-the-counter antihistamines like diphenhydramine (Benadryl) are commonly used to treat mild allergic reactions, so it's a logical leap to think they might also work for severe reactions. Media portrayals sometimes simplify the treatment of allergic reactions, reinforcing this belief.

Reality

Anaphylaxis requires immediate administration of epinephrine. Over-the-counter antihistamines are not effective for treating severe allergic reactions.

When Anaphylaxis Occurs

Anaphylaxis can be triggered by foods, insect stings, medications, or other allergens. Symptoms include difficulty breathing, swelling of the face and throat, hives, rapid pulse, and loss of consciousness. This is a medical emergency that requires immediate treatment.

Why This Thought is Correct

Epinephrine is the only effective treatment for anaphylaxis as it works quickly to reverse the severe symptoms. Antihistamines do not act fast enough or with enough potency to treat the life-threatening aspects of anaphylaxis.

What You Can Do in That Situation

Steps to Handle Anaphylaxis

1. **Call Emergency Services:** Immediately dial 911 or your local emergency number.

2. **Administer Epinephrine (if available):** If the person has an epinephrine auto-injector ("EpiPen"), and help them use it (instructions below).

    A) Locate and retrieve the EpiPen. It is typically stored in a plastic carrying case.

    B) Take the EpiPen out of its protective case.

    C) Hold the EpiPen with your dominant hand and remove the blue safety cap by pulling it straight up. This will activate the device.

    D) **Proper Positioning of the EpiPen**
       - **Hold the EpiPen:** Grip the EpiPen firmly in your dominant hand with the

orange tip (needle end) pointing
downward.

- **Select the Injection Site:** The
recommended injection site is the outer
thigh, halfway between the knee and the
hip. The EpiPen can be administered
through clothing if necessary.

E) **Administering the Injection**

- **Press and Hold:** Place the orange tip
against the outer thigh at a right angle (90
degrees) to the leg. Push the EpiPen
firmly into the thigh until you hear a
click. This indicates that the injection has
started.
- **Hold for 3 Seconds:** Keep the EpiPen
pressed against the thigh for a full 3
seconds to ensure the entire dose is
delivered.

F) **Withdraw the EpiPen** by pulling it straight
out of the thigh. The orange tip will
automatically extend to cover the needle.

G) **Massage the Injection Site:** Gently
massage the injection site for about 10
seconds to help disperse the medication.

3. **Monitor the Person**

- **Stay with the Person:** Keep them calm and lying down. If they feel faint, elevate their legs.
- **Monitor Symptoms:** Watch for signs of improvement or worsening. If symptoms persist, a second dose may be administered with a new EpiPen, if available, but should be reserved for instructions from the healthcare professionals. **Remember that the symptoms may improve for a short while and return, which is why monitoring is crucial**

4. **Dispose of the EpiPen**

- **Safely Dispose:** Place the used EpiPen back into its carrying case and give it to emergency responders for proper disposal. Do not throw it away in regular trash.

Important Points to Remember

- **Use Promptly:** Administer the EpiPen at the first sign of a severe allergic reaction. Delaying treatment can reduce single dose efficacy, and can lead to serious complications.

- **Correct Positioning:** Always use the outer thigh as the injection site. Do not inject into the buttocks, hands, feet, or other parts of the body.

- **Hold for 3 Seconds:** Ensure you hold the EpiPen in place for at least 3 seconds to deliver the full dose.

- **Seek Medical Help:** <u>Always</u> seek professional medical assistance after using an EpiPen, as symptoms of anaphylaxis can recur.

Emotional Support and Communication

- **Stay Calm and Reassuring:** Speak in a calm and supportive manner to help the person remain calm. Explain that help is on the way and that the epinephrine will help.
- **Provide Continuous Support:** Stay with the person, offering comfort and reassurance until emergency medical personnel arrive.

Diabetic Ketoacidosis (DKA)

Misconception

Give insulin immediately to a person suspected of DKA.

When and How This Misconception Could Occur

This misconception often occurs in situations where someone with diabetes experiences symptoms of hyperglycemia, and well-meaning bystanders think administering insulin will quickly resolve the issue. It can happen in environments where there is limited understanding of diabetic emergencies, such as schools, workplaces, or public spaces.

Why This Thought is Popular

The idea stems from the general knowledge that insulin lowers blood sugar, so it seems logical to administer it during a hyperglycemic crisis. Popular media and anecdotal advice might reinforce this belief, leading people to act without fully understanding the condition's complexities.

Reality

DKA requires professional medical treatment. Do not administer insulin unless directed by a healthcare provider. Seek emergency medical help as soon as possible.

When DKA Occurs

DKA is a serious complication of diabetes that can occur when the body starts breaking down fats at an excessive rate, producing ketones, which make the blood more acidic.

It can result from insulin deficiency, infection, illness, or severe stress. Symptoms include high blood sugar, excessive thirst, frequent urination, nausea, abdominal pain, weakness, and confusion.

Why This Thought is Correct

Administering insulin without proper medical supervision can be dangerous. The individual needs a controlled environment where their electrolyte levels and overall condition can be monitored. Immediate professional medical treatment is crucial to manage the complexity of DKA effectively and safely.

What You Can Do in That Situation

Steps to Handle Suspected DKA

1. **Recognize the Symptoms:** Look for signs of DKA such as extreme thirst, frequent urination, nausea, vomiting, abdominal pain, weakness, and confusion. The person may also have a fruity smell on their breath.

2. **Check for Medical Identification:** Determine if the person has diabetes by looking for medical identification jewelry or cards.

3. **Do Not Give Insulin:** Avoid administering insulin unless explicitly directed by a healthcare professional. Incorrect dosing can lead to severe complications.

4. **Provide Fluids:** If the person is conscious and able to swallow, provide sips of water to prevent dehydration. Do not give sugary drinks.

5. **Seek Emergency Help:** Call emergency services immediately. Inform them of the person's symptoms and that they have diabetes.

6. **Monitor the Person:** Keep the person comfortable and monitor their condition. Be prepared to provide information to medical responders when they arrive.

Emotional Support and Communication

- **Stay Calm and Reassuring:** Speak in a calm and soothing manner to reduce anxiety. Let the person know help is on the way and that they will be taken care of.
- **Explain Your Actions:** If they are conscious, explain what you are doing to keep them informed and less anxious.
- **Provide Continuous Support:** Stay with the person, offering comfort and reassurance until medical help arrives. Your presence and calm demeanor can significantly help in managing their stress and fear.

Chapter 2: Traumatic Injuries

In this chapter, we will be shifting the focus to traumatic injuries. Whether from accidents or violent encounters, these situations often happen when least expected. The ability to manage severe bleeding, stabilize fractures, and provide first aid for gunshot and stab wounds can be crucial in preventing further harm and saving lives.

This chapter covers the essential first aid techniques for handling these types of traumatic injuries, equipping you with the knowledge to respond confidently and competently. By mastering these skills, you become a critical first responder capable of making a significant impact in emergency situations.

Gunshot Wound

Misconception

Attempt to remove the bullet from the wound.

When and How This Misconception Could Occur

This misconception might arise in situations where people are trying to stop the damage caused by a gunshot wound, thinking that removing the bullet will prevent further harm. It can occur in any setting where a shooting has taken place.

Why This Thought is Popular

Movies and TV shows often dramatize the removal of bullets, making it seem like a crucial step in first aid. The idea that the bullet is the main cause of damage and should be removed immediately can be misleading.

Reality

Do not attempt to remove the bullet. Control the bleeding and seek immediate medical help.

When Gunshot Wounds Occur

Gunshot wounds can occur from accidents, violent encounters, or self-inflicted harm. They pose significant risks due to potential damage to internal organs and major blood vessels, leading to severe bleeding and other complications.

Why This Thought is Correct

Removing the bullet can cause more harm by increasing bleeding and tissue damage. The priority should be to control the bleeding and stabilize the victim until professional medical help arrives.

What You Can Do in That Situation

Steps to Provide First Aid for a Gunshot Wound

1. **Ensure Personal Safety:** Check that the area is safe to approach. Ensure there are no immediate threats to your safety or the victim's safety.

2. **Call Emergency Services:** Contact emergency services and provide detailed information about the situation, including the location, number of victims, and the nature of their injuries.

3. **Assess the Victim:** Determine the victim's level of consciousness. Check for responsiveness and breathing. If the victim is unresponsive and not breathing, begin CPR.

4. **Control the Bleeding:** Apply direct pressure to the wound using a clean cloth, bandage, or your hand. Use enough pressure to stop or reduce the bleeding. If the bleeding is severe and cannot be controlled with direct pressure, consider applying a tourniquet if the wound is on a limb.

5. **Apply a Tourniquet (if necessary):** Place the tourniquet above the wound, closer to the torso. Tighten the tourniquet until the bleeding stops.

Note the time the tourniquet was applied and inform emergency responders upon their arrival.

6. **Seal Chest Wounds:** If the gunshot wound is to the chest, cover it with a piece of plastic or a sterile, non-porous material to prevent air from entering the chest cavity. Tape the material on three sides to create a one-way valve. This helps prevent a collapsed lung (tension pneumothorax).

7. **Prevent Shock:** Lay the victim flat on their back and elevate their legs about 12 inches, unless this causes pain or the victim has a head, neck, or back injury. Keep the victim warm with blankets or clothing. Reassure and comfort the victim to keep them as calm as possible.

8. **Monitor Vital Signs:** Continuously monitor the victim's breathing, pulse, and level of consciousness. Be prepared to perform CPR if the victim stops breathing or loses their pulse.

9. **Provide Information to Emergency Responders:** When emergency services arrive, provide them with all relevant information, including the location of the wound, any first aid administered, and the time the tourniquet was applied (if used).

Emotional Support and Communication

- **Stay Reassuring:** Speak in a calm, steady voice to reassure the injured person. Acknowledge their pain and fear, offering comfort and support.
- **Explain Your Actions:** Clearly explain what you are doing to help them understand and reduce their anxiety.
- **Maintain Eye Contact:** If they are conscious, maintain eye contact and provide continuous verbal reassurance to keep them focused and calm.

Stab Wound

Misconception

Remove the object from a stab wound.

When and How This Misconception Could Occur

In emergencies, there is a common impulse to remove a foreign object from the body, thinking it will stop further injury or contamination. This misconception can occur during accidents, violent incidents, or any situation involving impalement by an object.

Why This Thought is Popular

People often believe that the object is the source of damage and removing it will alleviate the problem. This notion is sometimes reinforced by dramatic representations in media where characters pull out objects heroically without apparent consequences.

Reality

Do not remove the object as it may be controlling bleeding. Stabilize the object and seek emergency medical help. For severe lacerations, apply direct pressure to control bleeding and seek medical assistance.

When Stab Wounds Occur

Stab wounds can happen due to accidents, falls, or violent encounters. They pose significant risks due to potential damage to internal organs and major blood vessels, leading to severe bleeding and other complications.

Why This Thought is Correct

The object may act as a plug, controlling bleeding and preventing further internal injury. Removing it can exacerbate bleeding and worsen the injury. Properly stabilizing the object and seeking immediate medical help is crucial for minimizing damage and increasing the chances of recovery.

What You Can Do in That Situation

Steps to Handle Stab Wounds and Severe Lacerations

1. **Assess the Injury:** Determine the severity of the wound. If there is an object embedded, do not attempt to remove it.

2. **Stabilize the Object:** Use bulky dressings or clothing to stabilize the object, preventing it from moving and causing further injury.

3. **Apply Pressure (for Lacerations):** For severe lacerations without embedded objects, apply direct pressure using a clean cloth or bandage to control bleeding.

4. **Elevate the Limb:** If possible, elevate the injured limb above the level of the heart to reduce bleeding.

5. **Seek Emergency Help:** Call emergency services immediately. Provide clear information about the injury and follow their guidance until help arrives.

6. **Monitor Vital Signs:** Keep the person calm and monitor their breathing, consciousness, and circulation. Be prepared to perform CPR if necessary.

Emotional Support and Communication

- **Stay Reassuring:** Speak in a calm, steady voice to reassure the injured person. Acknowledge their pain and fear, offering comfort and support.
- **Explain Your Actions:** Clearly explain what you are doing to help them understand and reduce their anxiety.
- **Maintain Eye Contact:** If they are conscious, maintain eye contact and provide continuous verbal reassurance to keep them focused and calm.

Severe Lacerations

Misconception

Minor cuts don't require medical attention.

When and How This Misconception Could Occur

In everyday life, people might downplay the severity of cuts, thinking they can handle them with basic first aid. This misconception can occur in homes, workplaces, or any setting where minor injuries are common.

Why This Thought is Popular

The idea that minor cuts can be managed without professional help stems from the belief that as long as the bleeding stops, the injury will heal on its own. People might not realize the risk of infection or the need for proper wound care.

Reality

Severe lacerations can cause significant blood loss and may require professional medical treatment.

When Slicing Injuries Occur

Slicing injuries can result from accidents with sharp objects, self-inflicted harm, or violent encounters. These injuries can range from minor cuts to deep lacerations affecting muscles, tendons, or blood vessels.

Why This Thought is Correct

Proper wound care is crucial to prevent infection and promote healing. Even seemingly minor cuts can become serious if not treated correctly. Severe lacerations need medical evaluation to ensure there is no underlying damage and to provide appropriate treatment.

What You Can Do in That Situation

Steps to Handle Severe Lacerations

1. **Assess the Situation:** Ensure the area is safe to approach. Call emergency services if the laceration is severe.

2. **Control Bleeding:** Apply direct pressure to the wound using a clean cloth or bandage. Maintain pressure until the bleeding stops. If blood soaks through the cloth, add more layers without removing the original cloth.

3. **Elevate the Wound:** If the wound is on a limb, elevate it above the level of the heart to reduce bleeding.

4. **Clean the Wound (if minor):** For less severe cuts, rinse the wound with clean water to remove debris. Avoid using hydrogen peroxide or alcohol as they can damage tissue.

5. **Apply a Clean Dressing:** Cover the wound with a sterile dressing or clean cloth. Secure it with tape or bandages.

6. **Monitor for Shock:** Lay the victim flat on their back and elevate their legs about 12 inches if possible. Keep the victim warm and calm to reduce the risk of shock.

7. **Seek Medical Attention:** For severe lacerations, seek immediate medical attention. Even minor cuts may need professional care to prevent infection and ensure proper healing.

Emotional Support and Communication

- **Stay Reassuring:** Speak in a calm, steady voice to reassure the injured person. Acknowledge their pain and fear, offering comfort and support.
- **Explain Your Actions:** Clearly explain what you are doing to help them understand and reduce their anxiety.
- **Maintain Eye Contact:** If they are conscious, maintain eye contact and provide continuous verbal reassurance to keep them focused and calm.

<u>Burns</u>

Misconception

Apply ice or butter to a burn.

When and How This Misconception Could Occur

This misconception often arises in households where first aid knowledge is based on passed-down advice rather than medical training. It can occur in kitchens, workplaces, or outdoor settings where burns from heat, chemicals, or sun exposure happen.

Why This Thought is Popular

Rubbing the affected area might seem logical because friction generates heat, and it's a common reaction to feeling cold. Historical practices and survival myths can also perpetuate this idea.

Reality

Run cool (not cold) water over the burn for 10-20 minutes, cover with a clean, non-stick bandage, and seek medical help for severe burns. Do not apply ice, butter, or any ointments.

When Burns Occur

Burns can occur from direct contact with heat, chemicals, electricity, or radiation. Common scenarios include kitchen accidents, chemical spills, sunburns, or electrical malfunctions. The severity of burns ranges from minor (first-degree) to severe (third-degree).

Why This Thought is Correct

Cool water helps reduce the temperature of the burn and prevents further tissue damage. Ice can cause frostbite and further damage the skin, while butter or ointments can trap heat, increasing tissue damage and infection risk. Proper burn care involves cooling the burn, protecting it, and seeking medical help if needed.

What You Can Do in That Situation

Steps to Treat Burns

1. **Stop the Burning Process:** Remove the person from the source of the burn. For electrical burns, ensure the power is off before touching the person.

2. **Cool the Burn:** Run cool (not cold) water over the burn for 10-20 minutes. This helps reduce pain and swelling.

3. **Cover the Burn:** Use a clean, non-stick bandage or cloth to cover the burn. Avoid using cotton balls or anything that can stick to the burn.

4. **Do Not Apply Ice or Butter:** Avoid home remedies like ice, butter, or ointments. They can cause more harm than good.

5. **Seek Medical Help:** For severe burns (blistering, deep burns, or burns covering large areas), seek immediate medical attention.

Emotional Support and Communication

- **Stay Calm and Reassuring:** Speak softly and calmly to the person. Let them know that you are helping and that they will be okay.
- **Explain Your Actions:** Inform them of what you are doing and why it helps. This can ease their anxiety and help them follow instructions.
- **Provide Continuous Support:** Stay with the person, offering comfort and reassurance until the bleeding stops or help arrives.

<u>Broken Bone</u>
(Fracture)

When to Perform Emergency First Aid

Suspect a fracture if there is intense pain, swelling, visible deformity, or inability to use the limb.

What You Can Do in That Situation

Steps to Take

1. **Immobilize the Injury:** Do not try to realign the bone. Use splints or improvised materials (e.g., sticks and cloth) to immobilize the affected area.

2. **Apply a Cold Pack:** Use a cold pack or ice wrapped in cloth to reduce swelling and pain.

3. **Elevate the Limb:** If possible, elevate the injured limb to reduce swelling.

4. **Seek Medical Help:** Call 911 or take the person to the nearest emergency room.

<u>Eye Injury</u>

When to Perform Emergency First Aid

Eye injuries can include chemical exposure, foreign objects, cuts, and blows to the eye.

What You Can Do in That Situation

Steps to Take

1. **Chemical Exposure:**
   - Rinse the eye with clean water for at least 15 minutes.
   - Hold the eye open while flushing.
   - Seek immediate medical help.

2. **Foreign Object:**
   - Do not rub the eye.
   - Rinse the eye with clean water or saline solution.
   - If the object is embedded, cover the eye with a clean cloth and seek medical help.

3. **Cuts or Blows:**
   - Cover the eye with a clean cloth or eye shield.
   - Seek immediate medical attention.

Chapter 3: Environmental Emergencies

Environmental emergencies tend to be things such as hypothermia and heatstroke, things that result from extreme weather conditions and environmental factors. These situations can be life-threatening if not addressed promptly and correctly.

This chapter explores the critical steps needed to prevent and respond to such emergencies, providing you with the knowledge to protect yourself and others from the dangers of the environment.

By staying informed and prepared, you can navigate these challenges with confidence and care.

Heat Exhaustion and Heat Stroke

When to Perform Emergency First Aid

Symptoms of heat exhaustion include heavy sweating, weakness, cold, pale skin, and nausea. Heat stroke symptoms include hot, dry skin, high body temperature, confusion, and loss of consciousness.

What You Can Do in That Situation

Steps to Take

1. **Move to a Cooler Place:** Get the person out of the heat and into a cooler environment.

2. **Hydrate:** Give the person small sips of cool water if they are conscious and able to drink.

3. **Cool the Body:**
   - Apply cool, wet cloths to the skin or use a cool bath.
   - Fan the person to promote evaporation.

4. **Seek Medical Help:** Call 911 if symptoms worsen or if you suspect heat stroke.

<u>Hypothermia</u>

When to Perform Emergency First Aid

Symptoms include shivering, slurred speech, slow breathing, and confusion.

What You Can Do in That Situation

Steps to Take

1. **Move to a Warm Place:** Get the person out of the cold and into a warmer environment.

2. **Remove Wet Clothing:** Replace with dry, warm clothing.

3. **Warm the Body:** Use blankets, warm water bottles, or body heat to warm the person gradually.

4. **Provide Warm Drinks:** Offer warm, non-alcoholic beverages if the person is conscious.

5. **Seek Medical Help:** Call 911 for severe hypothermia cases.

Frostbite

Misconception

Rub the affected area to warm it.

When and How This Misconception Could Occur

This misconception often arises in cold environments, such as during outdoor activities in winter or in settings where someone is exposed to freezing temperatures without adequate protection. It can occur among those unfamiliar with proper cold injury first aid.

Why This Thought is Popular

Rubbing the affected area might seem logical because friction generates heat, and it's a common reaction to feeling cold. Historical practices and survival myths can also perpetuate this idea.

Reality

Do not rub frostbitten skin. Move to a warm place, use warm (not hot) water to gradually warm the area, and seek medical attention.

When Frostbite Occurs

Frostbite occurs when skin and underlying tissues freeze due to prolonged exposure to cold temperatures. It commonly affects extremities like fingers, toes, ears, and the nose. Symptoms include numbness, tingling, and skin discoloration.

Why This Thought is Correct

Rubbing frostbitten skin can cause further damage by breaking delicate tissues and ice crystals within the skin. Proper rewarming techniques prevent additional injury and promote better recovery.

What You Can Do in That Situation

Steps to Treat Frostbite

1. **Move to a Warm Place:** Get the person out of the cold and into a warmer environment as soon as possible.

2. **Remove Wet Clothing:** Take off any wet clothing and replace it with dry, warm garments to prevent further heat loss.

3. **Gradual Rewarming:** Submerge the affected area in warm (not hot) water, around 99-104°F (37-40°C), for 15-30 minutes. Avoid using direct heat sources like stoves or heating pads.

4. **Protect the Skin:** Do not rub or massage the frostbitten area. Instead, handle it gently to prevent further damage.

5. **Cover with Clean Bandages:** After rewarming, cover the area with clean, dry bandages. Place gauze between fingers or toes to prevent them from sticking together.

6. **Seek Medical Attention:** Frostbite requires professional medical evaluation. Severe cases may need hospitalization and further treatment.

Emotional Support and Communication

- **Stay Calm and Reassuring:** Speak calmly and reassuringly to help the person remain calm. Explain each step you are taking.
- **Monitor for Hypothermia:** Check for signs of hypothermia, such as shivering, confusion, or drowsiness, and take appropriate action if needed.
- **Provide Continuous Support:** Stay with the person, offering comfort and reassurance until they are warm and medical help is available.

Chapter 4: General Emergencies

We can now look into the more average everyday incidents, such as burns, nosebleeds, and choking. These are the types of emergencies that can almost be labeled as common occurrences, but have the ability to escalate into much more serious emergencies if not handled properly.

This chapter provides practical guidance on managing these incidents with ease and precision. By understanding the correct first aid responses and debunking common misconceptions, you can ensure the safety and well-being of yourself and others in everyday situations.

These skills are not just useful; they are essential for maintaining a safe environment in daily life.

<u>Choking</u>

Misconception

Perform the Heimlich maneuver on a person who is coughing.

When and How This Misconception Could Occur

This misconception often arises in dining settings, workplaces, or homes where someone experiences difficulty swallowing. People might panic and think that any sign of choking, including coughing, requires the Heimlich maneuver.

Why This Thought is Popular

The Heimlich maneuver is widely taught as the primary response to choking, but the distinction between mild and severe airway obstruction is often misunderstood. Media portrayals can also contribute to this misconception by showing the Heimlich maneuver performed at the slightest sign of choking.

Reality

If the person is coughing or can speak, allow them to try to expel the object. If they cannot breathe, cough, or speak, perform the Heimlich maneuver.

When Choking Occurs

Choking happens when an object blocks the airway, preventing normal breathing. It can occur while eating, especially with improperly chewed food, or when small objects are accidentally inhaled. Recognizing the severity of choking is critical for appropriate response.

Why This Thought is Correct

Coughing is a natural reflex that can often dislodge an object without intervention. Performing the Heimlich maneuver prematurely can cause unnecessary harm or panic. It is essential to assess the situation correctly and act only when the airway is severely obstructed.

What You Can Do in That Situation

Steps to Help Someone Who is Choking

1. **Assess the Severity:** Determine if the person can breathe, speak, or cough. If they are coughing forcefully, encourage them to continue as this may dislodge the object.

2. **Do Not Intervene Prematurely:** Allow the person to try to expel the object on their own if they are able to cough or speak.

3. **Perform the Heimlich Maneuver:** If the person cannot breathe, cough, or speak, and is making the universal choking sign (hands around the throat):

   - Stand behind the person and wrap your arms around their waist.
   - Make a fist with one hand and place it just above their navel.

- Grasp your fist with the other hand and perform quick, inward and upward thrusts.
- Continue until the object is expelled or the person becomes unconscious.

4. **Seek Emergency Help:** Call 911 immediately if the person is unable to expel the object.

For Unconscious Choking Victims

1. **Lower the Person to the Ground:** Carefully lay the person on their back.

2. **Begin CPR:** Start chest compressions and look for the object in the mouth after each set of compressions. Remove the object if visible and accessible.

3. **Continue Until Help Arrives:** Perform CPR until the object is expelled or emergency medical personnel arrive.

Emotional Support and Communication

- **Stay Calm and Reassuring:** Maintain a calm demeanor to prevent further panic. Speak in a clear and reassuring manner.
- **Encourage Self-Help:** If the person is coughing, encourage them to keep trying to cough out the object while you stay close by.

- **Provide Continuous Support:** Stay with the person, offering verbal comfort and physical presence until the situation is resolved.

<u>Poisoning</u>

Misconception

Induce vomiting after swallowing poison

When and How This Misconception Could Occur

This misconception can occur in households, especially where children or pets accidentally ingest toxic substances. It might also happen in workplaces with exposure to chemicals. The idea to induce vomiting might arise from panic and the instinct to expel the harmful substance quickly.

Why This Thought is Popular

The belief that inducing vomiting removes the poison from the body is based on the logical but flawed notion that immediate expulsion reduces harm. This idea has been passed down through generations and reinforced by outdated first aid practices.

Reality

Do not induce vomiting unless directed by poison control or a healthcare professional. Call poison control immediately and follow their instructions.

When Poisoning Occurs

Poisoning can happen from ingesting household chemicals, medications, toxic plants, or contaminated food. Symptoms vary widely depending on the substance but can include nausea, vomiting, abdominal pain, difficulty breathing, and altered mental state.

Why This Thought is Correct

Inducing vomiting can cause further damage by exposing the esophagus and mouth to the poison again. Some substances can cause burns or other injuries on their way back up. Proper management involves contacting poison control or seeking medical help to get the right guidance.

What You Can Do in That Situation

Steps to Handle Poisoning

1. **Call Poison Control:** Contact poison control immediately at 1-800-222-1222 in the U.S. or the local equivalent in other countries. Provide detailed information about the substance ingested and follow their instructions.

2. **Do Not Induce Vomiting:** Avoid giving anything by mouth unless instructed by poison control or a healthcare professional.

3. **Check for Symptoms:** Monitor the person for symptoms like difficulty breathing, drowsiness, or changes in behavior.

4. **Move to Fresh Air:** If the poisoning is due to inhalation, move the person to fresh air immediately.

5. **Remove Contaminated Clothing:** If the poison is on the skin or clothing, remove contaminated clothing and rinse the skin with water for at least 15 minutes.

6. **Seek Emergency Help:** If the person shows severe symptoms or if poison control advises, seek immediate medical attention.

Emotional Support and Communication

- **Stay Calm and Reassuring:** Speak in a calm and composed manner to keep the person from panicking. Explain that help is on the way.

- **Provide Clear Instructions:** Follow poison control's instructions carefully and relay them clearly to anyone assisting you.

- **Offer Continuous Support:** Stay with the person, offering comfort and reassurance until professional help arrives or the situation is under control.

Nosebleeds

Misconception

Tilt the head back during a nosebleed.

When and How This Misconception Could Occur

This misconception can occur in any setting where a nosebleed happens, such as schools, sports events, or at home. It often arises from an instinct to prevent blood from spilling out and to keep the person looking presentable.

Why This Thought is Popular

The advice to tilt the head back is a natural response to prevent blood from making a mess. It's also a common myth perpetuated by outdated first aid practices and media portrayals, where characters are often shown tilting their heads back during a nosebleed.

Reality

Sit up straight and lean slightly forward. Pinch the soft part of your nose and maintain pressure for 10-15 minutes. Avoid lying down or tilting the head back.

When Nosebleeds Occur

Nosebleeds can be caused by dry air, nose picking, allergies, infections, or trauma to the nose. They are common in children but can occur at any age. While usually not serious, they can be alarming and uncomfortable.

Why This Thought is Correct

Tilting the head back can cause blood to flow down the throat, leading to choking or vomiting. Leaning forward prevents blood from entering the throat and allows it to exit through the nostrils, which is safer and more hygienic.

What You Can Do in That Situation

Steps to Treat Nosebleeds

1. **Sit Up Straight and Lean Forward:** This helps keep blood from running down the throat and aids in blood drainage through the nose.

2. **Pinch the Nose:** Pinch the soft part of the nose just below the bony bridge. Apply steady pressure for 10-15 minutes without checking to see if the bleeding has stopped.

3. **Breathe Through the Mouth:** Encourage the person to breathe through their mouth while pinching their nose.

4. **Avoid Lying Down or Tilting the Head Back:** Keep the head elevated and leaning forward.

5. **Apply a Cold Compress:** Place a cold compress or ice pack on the bridge of the nose to help constrict blood vessels and reduce bleeding.

6. **Seek Medical Help if Necessary:** If bleeding persists for more than 20 minutes or occurs frequently, seek medical advice.

Emotional Support and Communication

- **Stay Calm and Reassuring:** Speak in a calm and comforting manner. Let the person know that nosebleeds are common and usually not serious.

- **Explain Your Actions:** Inform them of what you are doing and why it helps. This can ease their anxiety and help them follow instructions.

- **Provide Continuous Support:** Stay with the person, offering comfort and reassurance until the bleeding stops or help arrives.

Chapter 5: Emergency Procedures
and
Essential Techniques

Mastering essential first aid techniques is the cornerstone of effective emergency response. This chapter focuses on key skills such as CPR, using an AED, administering an EpiPen, and emergency suturing.

These techniques are vital for stabilizing victims and providing life-saving care until professional help arrives. By learning and practicing these methods, you enhance your ability to act decisively in emergencies, making a meaningful difference in critical situations.

Applying a Tourniquet

Misconception

You should never use a tourniquet because it will cause the loss of the limb.

When and How This Misconception Could Occur

This misconception is pervasive and often rooted in outdated medical advice and dramatized portrayals in media. People might recall stories from wartime or historical accounts where tourniquets were misapplied, leading to severe complications or amputations. The fear of causing irreversible damage can lead to hesitation or refusal to use a tourniquet when it's genuinely needed.

Why This Thought is Popular

The idea that a tourniquet leads to limb loss comes from historical contexts where medical knowledge and resources were limited. In the past, improper use or prolonged application of tourniquets did result in significant harm. These stories have persisted and been amplified by movies and TV shows, reinforcing the belief that tourniquets are dangerous.

Reality

In severe bleeding situations where direct pressure fails, a tourniquet can be life-saving.

When to Use a Tourniquet

Tourniquets should be used in scenarios of severe arterial bleeding where direct pressure is insufficient to stop the flow. This can occur in situations like:

- Deep cuts or lacerations from accidents.
- Severe injuries in remote locations where immediate medical help is unavailable.
- During mass casualty incidents where resources are limited, and bleeding control is critical.

Why This Thought is Correct

Modern medical guidelines emphasize the correct application of tourniquets as a critical intervention to prevent exsanguination (bleeding out). When applied correctly and monitored, a tourniquet can control life-threatening bleeding until professional medical help is available. Advances in medical technology and better training have improved the safety and effectiveness of tourniquets.

What You Can Do in That Situation

Steps to Apply a Tourniquet

1. **Assess the Situation:** Ensure that using a tourniquet is necessary. Look for severe, uncontrollable bleeding.

2. **Position the Tourniquet:** Place the tourniquet 2-3 inches above the wound, avoiding joints. If the wound is on the lower limb, apply it above the knee; for the upper limb, above the elbow.

3. **Tighten the Tourniquet:** Pull the strap tightly and secure it. Use the windlass (a rod or stick used to twist the tourniquet) to tighten until the bleeding stops. It will be painful for the injured person, but this indicates proper application.

4. **Secure the Windlass:** Once the bleeding has stopped, secure the windlass to prevent it from unwinding.

5. **Note the Time:** Write the time of application on the tourniquet or the person's skin. Medical professionals need to know how long it has been in place.

6. **Monitor and Seek Help:** Do not remove the tourniquet. Keep the person calm and seek immediate medical assistance. Inform emergency responders about the tourniquet and the time of application.

Emotional Support and Communication

- **Stay Calm:** Your composure can help keep the injured person calm. Explain what you are doing and why it's necessary.
- **Reassure Them** that the tourniquet is a temporary measure to control bleeding and help is on the way.
- **Monitor Their Condition:** Keep an eye on their overall condition, ensuring they remain conscious and responsive. Comfort them through the pain and fear by maintaining a steady, reassuring tone.

<u>Using a Defibrillator</u>

How to Use an Automated External Defibrillator (AED) - Portable Device

Step-by-Step Instructions for Portable AED

1. Assess the Situation

- Ensure the area is safe for you and the victim.
- Check for responsiveness and breathing. If the person is unresponsive and not breathing or not breathing normally, call 911 or your local emergency number and get the AED.

2. Turn On the AED

- Open the AED case and turn on the device by pressing the power button or lifting the lid, depending on the model.

3. Attach the Pads

- Expose the person's chest and ensure it is dry.
- Attach the AED pads to the person's bare chest. Place one pad on the upper right side of the chest (just below the collarbone) and the other pad on the lower left side of the chest (a few inches below the armpit).

4. Analyze the Heart Rhythm

- Follow the AED's voice prompts. The device will instruct you to stay clear of the person while it analyzes the heart rhythm.

- Ensure no one is touching the person during the analysis.

5. Deliver the Shock

- If the AED advises a shock, ensure everyone is clear of the person and press the shock button when prompted.
- The AED will administer the shock automatically in some models; ensure you follow the specific device's instructions.

6. Perform CPR

- After the shock is delivered, or if no shock is advised, start CPR immediately. Provide chest compressions and rescue breaths as instructed by the AED until emergency medical personnel arrive or the person shows signs of life.

7. Continue Following AED Prompts

- The AED will continue to monitor the heart rhythm and may prompt you to deliver additional shocks or continue CPR.
- Follow the device's prompts until professional help arrives or the person recovers.

How to Use a Hospital Defibrillator - Manual Defibrillator

Step-by-Step Instructions for Manual Defibrillator

1. Assess the Situation

- Ensure the area is safe for you and the patient.
- Check for responsiveness and breathing. If the patient is unresponsive and not breathing or not breathing normally, call for help and initiate CPR while preparing the defibrillator.

2. Prepare the Defibrillator

- Turn on the manual defibrillator by pressing the power button.
- Select the appropriate energy level based on hospital protocols (typically 120-200 joules for biphasic defibrillators and 360 joules for monophasic defibrillators).

3. Attach the Pads

- Expose the patient's chest and ensure it is dry.
- Attach the defibrillator pads to the patient's bare chest. Place one pad on the upper right side of the chest (just below the collarbone) and the other pad on the lower left side of the chest (a few inches below the armpit).

4. Charge the Defibrillator

- Press the charge button to charge the defibrillator

to the selected energy level.

5. Ensure Safety

- Ensure everyone is clear of the patient. Loudly announce "Clear!" and visually confirm that no one is touching the patient or the bed.

6. Deliver the Shock

- Press the shock button to deliver the electrical shock to the patient's heart.

7. Continue Resuscitation

- Immediately resume CPR for 2 minutes (or as per hospital protocol) after delivering the shock.
- Reassess the patient's rhythm and condition after 2 minutes of CPR. If the patient remains in a shockable rhythm, repeat the defibrillation process.

8. Follow Protocols

- Continue to follow hospital resuscitation protocols and use the defibrillator as needed until the patient regains a normal rhythm or is declared otherwise by medical personnel.

Key Points to Remember

- **Safety First:** Always ensure the area is safe and no one is touching the patient during the defibrillation process.
- **Proper Pad Placement:** Correct placement of the pads is crucial for effective defibrillation.

- Follow Prompts: Both AEDs and manual defibrillators provide prompts and guidelines. Follow these carefully.
- Immediate CPR: Combine defibrillation with CPR to maximize the chances of survival.

<u>Emergency Tracheotomy</u>

When to Perform an Emergency Tracheotomy

An emergency tracheotomy (more accurately called a cricothyrotomy in this context) is a last-resort procedure used when all other methods to clear an airway have failed. This procedure should only be performed when the person cannot breathe due to a complete airway obstruction and is at imminent risk of death. Situations might include:

- Severe allergic reaction causing swelling (anaphylaxis) when epinephrine is unavailable or ineffective.
- Blockage of the airway by a foreign object that cannot be removed by other means (e.g., Heimlich maneuver).
- Trauma to the face or throat preventing normal breathing.

Risks and Considerations

- Risks: Infection, bleeding, damage to the vocal cords or thyroid gland, and long-term complications.
- Considerations: This is a high-risk procedure and should only be performed if immediate medical help is not available, and the person is in critical condition.

How to Perform an Emergency Tracheotomy with Household Supplies

Supplies Needed

- ❖ A sharp knife or razor blade (sterilized if possible)
- ❖ A hollow tube (e.g., the barrel of a ballpoint pen, a straw, or a similar object)
- ❖ Alcohol or antiseptic wipes (if available)
- ❖ Clean cloths or bandages

Steps to Perform the Procedure

1. Assess the Situation

- Ensure the person is unresponsive, not breathing, and all other airway clearance
- Call emergency services immediately.

2. Prepare the Area

- Find a clean area to work. If possible, use antiseptic wipes to clean the person's neck.
- Wash your hands or use hand sanitizer if available.

3. Locate the Cricothyroid Membrane

- The cricothyroid membrane is located in the neck, between the thyroid cartilage (Adam's apple) and the cricoid cartilage.
- Feel for the Adam's apple and move your fingers downward until you find a slight indentation or soft spot just below it.

4. Make the Incision

- Using the sharp knife or razor blade, make a horizontal incision about 1/2 to 3/4 inch.
- Be careful not to cut too deeply. The goal is to create an opening into the airway.

5. Insert the Tube

- Quickly insert the hollow tube into the incision you made.
- Ensure the tube is positioned correctly and air can pass through it. You should see the chest rise and fall if the tube is placed correctly.

6. Secure the Tube

- Once the tube is inserted, secure it with cloth or bandages to prevent it from moving.
- Ensure the airway remains open and check for proper airflow.

7. Monitor the Victim

- Keep the person as calm and still as possible. Monitor their breathing and be prepared to provide additional support if necessary.
- Wait for emergency medical personnel to arrive and take over.

Important Notes

- **Only as a Last Resort** This procedure is extremely risky and should only be attempted when all other methods have failed and death is imminent.

- **Medical Training:** Ideally, only individuals with medical training should perform this procedure. If untrained, attempt it only if absolutely necessary and with great caution.
- **Seek Immediate Help:** Always call for professional medical help before attempting this procedure.

Aftercare and Professional Medical Intervention

- Once emergency services arrive, inform them of the procedure performed.
- The person will need immediate hospital care to prevent complications and provide proper medical treatment.

<u>Reinflating a Collapsed Lung</u>

A collapsed lung, or pneumothorax, is a serious medical emergency often caused by chest trauma, such as a stab wound, that allows air to enter the pleural space. This can cause the lung to collapse and impair breathing. In an emergency situation where professional medical help is not immediately available, you may need to perform a needle decompression to relieve the pressure.

When to Perform Needle Decompression

- The person has a penetrating chest wound.

- Symptoms of a tension pneumothorax are present, such as severe difficulty breathing, rapid heart rate, low blood pressure, and distended neck veins.

- The person is showing signs of respiratory distress and you have no immediate access to professional medical help.

Supplies Needed

- A large-bore needle or catheter (14-gauge or larger, about 1.75 to 2 inches long)
- Alcohol or antiseptic wipes (if available)
- Sterile or clean cloths
- Tape or adhesive (optional)

Steps to Perform Needle Decompression

1. Ensure Safety and Call for Help

- **Ensure the Scene is Safe:** Make sure there is no ongoing threat to your safety.
- **Call Emergency Services:** Dial 911 or your local emergency number and provide detailed information about the situation.

2. Prepare the Equipment

- **Sterilize the Needle:** If possible, use alcohol or antiseptic wipes to sterilize the needle or catheter.

3. Locate the Insertion Site

- **Find the Correct Location:** The preferred site for needle decompression is the second intercostal space in the midclavicular line (roughly between the second and third rib, just below the collarbone).
- **Count Ribs:** Locate the clavicle (collarbone) and move down to the second rib. The intercostal space is just below this rib.
- **Midclavicular Line:** This is an imaginary line that runs vertically down from the midpoint of the clavicle.

4. Clean the Area

- **Clean the Skin:** If available, use alcohol or antiseptic wipes to clean the skin at the insertion site.

5. **Insert the Needle**

- **Position the Needle:** Hold the needle or catheter at a 90-degree angle to the chest wall.
- **Insert the Needle:** Insert the needle just above the third rib (to avoid the neurovascular bundle located below each rib) and advance it through the chest wall into the pleural space.
- **Feel for a "Pop":** You may feel a sudden decrease in resistance as the needle enters the pleural space.
- **Listen for Air Release:** If the needle is correctly placed, you should hear a rush of air as the trapped air is released, relieving the pressure on the lung.

6. **Secure the Needle (Optional)**

- **Secure the Needle:** If possible, secure the needle in place with tape or adhesive to prevent it from moving.

7. **Monitor the Victim**

- **Assess Breathing:** Check the person's breathing and watch for improvement in their respiratory status.
- **Reassure the Person:** Keep the person calm and still, and continue to monitor their condition until professional medical help arrives.

Aftercare

- **Seek Professional Medical Help:** Even if the needle decompression relieves the immediate symptoms, the person still needs urgent medical evaluation and treatment.

- **Inform Medical Personnel:** Provide details about the procedure, including the location and time of needle insertion, to the emergency responders.

Important Notes

- **High Risk:** Needle decompression is a high-risk procedure that can cause serious complications if not done correctly. It should only be performed in life-threatening situations when professional help is not immediately available.
- **Training:** Ideally, this procedure should be performed by someone with medical training. If untrained, proceed with extreme caution and follow instructions closely.

Understanding how to perform needle decompression can be life-saving in critical situations, but it is always preferable to seek professional medical help whenever possible. Proper knowledge and technique are essential to minimize risks and improve outcomes in emergency cases of a collapsed lung.

Emergency Suturing Technique with Household Supplies

When Sutures Are Needed

Suturing a wound may be necessary in an emergency to control bleeding and promote healing when professional medical help is not immediately available. Situations where sutures might be required include:

- Deep cuts or lacerations where the edges of the wound do not stay together on their own.

- Wounds that are longer than 1 inch.

- Wounds with continuous bleeding that cannot be controlled with pressure alone.

- Areas where the skin is under tension or frequently moves, such as joints or the face.

Supplies Needed

In the absence of a proper suture kit, you can use the following household items:

- Needle: A sewing needle (preferably sterilized)
- Thread: Strong, clean thread (e.g., dental floss, fishing line, or regular sewing thread)
- Sterilizing agent: Alcohol, boiling water, or flame to sterilize the needle and thread
- Clean cloth or bandages
- Scissors, a knife, or nail clippers (all sterilized)
- Antiseptic solution or clean water

❖ Tweezers (optional, sterilized if possible)

❖ Gloves (if available)

Steps to Perform Emergency Suturing

1. Ensure Safety and Call for Help

- **Ensure the Scene is Safe:** Make sure there is no ongoing threat to your safety.

- **Call Emergency Services:** Dial 911 or your local emergency number if possible, even if you attempt suturing.

2. Prepare the Equipment

Sterilize the Needle and Thread:

- **Needle:** Sterilize the needle by boiling it in water for at least 10 minutes, or by wiping it with alcohol and then passing it through a flame until it glows red. Allow it to cool before use.

- **Thread:** Sterilize the thread by soaking it in alcohol or boiling it with the needle.

3. Clean the Wound

- **Clean the Wound:** Rinse the wound thoroughly with clean water or an antiseptic solution to remove any debris or dirt.

- **Dry the Area:** Pat the area around the wound dry with a clean cloth or sterile gauze.

4. Assess the Wound

- **Determine the Need for Sutures:** Ensure that the wound meets the criteria for suturing. If in doubt, err on the side of caution and prepare to suture.

5. Prepare the Wound Edges

- Align the Wound Edges: Use clean fingers or sterilized tweezers to gently bring the edges of the wound together.

6. Begin Suturing

- **Thread the Needle:** Thread the sterilized needle with the sterilized thread and tie a knot approximately 2 inches from the end.
- **Start the First Stitch:**
  - Insert the needle approximately 0.5 cm (1/4 inch) from the edge of the wound.
  - Push the needle through the skin at a 90-degree angle and bring it up on the other side of the wound, again 0.5 cm (1/4 inch) from the edge.
- **Pull the Thread Through:** Gently pull the thread through the wound until the knot at the end stops it from going further.
  - If necessary, you can use the 2 inches of thread past the knot to tie a knot, but do so with caution to not overtighten, as the thread could cut through the skin or break itself.

7. Create Subsequent Stitches

- **Spacing:** Place each stitch about 0.5 cm (1/4 inch) apart, ensuring they are evenly spaced to hold the wound edges together securely.
- **Method:**
    - Repeat the stitching process, going from one side of the wound to the other, pulling the edges together with each stitch.
    - Ensure that each stitch is snug but not so tight that it causes the skin to pucker or cut into the flesh.

8. Finish the Suturing

- **End the Suturing:**
    - Once the wound is fully sutured, tie off the thread with a secure knot.
    - Cut the excess thread pieces, leaving a small tail to ensure the knot does not come undone.

9. Dress the Wound

- **Apply an Antiseptic:** Apply an antiseptic solution to the wound to reduce the risk of infection.
- **Cover the Wound:** Cover the sutured wound with a clean bandage or sterile gauze. Secure it with tape or a clean cloth. If on an active area, you can also run some tape strips perpendicularly across the wound to assist the stitches resistance to breaking.

10. **Monitor for Infection**

- **Signs of Infection:** Monitor the wound for signs of infection, such as redness, swelling, increased pain, warmth, or discharge.
- **Seek Medical Help:** Even if you have sutured the wound, seek professional medical evaluation and care as soon as possible to ensure proper healing and to address any complications.

Important Notes

- **Only as a Last Resort:** Suturing should only be performed in a life-threatening situation when professional medical help is not immediately available.
- **Proper Sterilization:** Ensure all equipment is as clean and sterile as possible to reduce the risk of infection.
- **Post-Suturing Care:** Keep the wound clean and dry, and monitor it closely until professional medical care is obtained.

Performing emergency suturing with household supplies is a high-risk procedure and should only be attempted when absolutely necessary. Proper technique and sterilization are essential to minimize the risk of infection and complications. Always seek professional medical help as soon as possible.

Chapter 6: Mnemonics for Emergency Situations

In the chaos of an emergency, quick recall of essential information can save lives. This chapter introduces useful mnemonics and quick reference guides that simplify complex procedures and ensure you remember crucial steps when it matters most.

These tools are designed to be easy to memorize and apply, providing you with a reliable resource for effective first aid. By incorporating these mnemonics into your first aid knowledge, you enhance your preparedness and ability to respond swiftly in any emergency.

Recognizing Stroke Symptoms: FAST

F - Face

Ask the person to smile. Does one side of the face droop?

- **What to Look For:** A lopsided or asymmetrical smile where one side of the face does not move as well as the other side.

- **Why It's Important:** Facial drooping is a common symptom of a stroke caused by muscle weakness or paralysis on one side of the body.

A - Arms

Ask the person to raise both arms. Does one arm drift downward?

- **What to Look For:** Difficulty lifting both arms to the same height, or one arm drifts downward or is unable to be raised.

- **Why It's Important:** Arm weakness or inability to raise an arm is another sign of muscle weakness due to a stroke.

S - Speech

Ask the person to repeat a simple phrase. Is their speech slurred or strange?

- **What to Look For:** Slurred, garbled, or difficult-to-understand speech. The person might also have trouble repeating a simple sentence correctly.

- **Why It's Important:** Speech difficulties are a hallmark of stroke, indicating potential damage to the areas of the brain responsible for language.

T - Time

If you observe any of these signs, it's time to call emergency services immediately.

- **What to Do:** Call 911 or your local emergency number without delay. Note the time when symptoms first appeared.

- **Why It's Important:** Time is critical in treating a stroke. The sooner the person receives medical treatment, the better their chances of reducing brain damage and improving recovery.

<u>Choking: ABC</u>
(Airway, Breathing, Circulation)

A - Airway

Ensure the person's airway is clear.

- **What to Do:** Ask if the person can speak or cough. If they can, encourage them to keep coughing to dislodge the object.

B - Breathing

Check for breathing difficulties.

- **What to Do:** If the person cannot breathe, perform the Heimlich maneuver.

C - Circulation

Monitor the person's circulation.

- **What to Do:** If the person becomes unconscious, begin CPR and call emergency services.

<u>Burns: COOL</u>
<u>(Cool, Over, Only, Loosely)</u>

C - Cool

Cool the burn with running water.

- **What to Do:** Run cool (not cold) water over the burn for 10-20 minutes.

O - Over

Cover the burn with a clean, non-stick dressing.

- **What to Do:** Use a sterile dressing or clean cloth to cover the burn.

O - Only

Only remove clothing and jewelry if not stuck to the burn.

- **What to Do:** Carefully remove any restrictive items around the burn area.

L - Loosely

Loosely cover the burn.

- **What to Do:** Ensure the dressing is not too tight to allow for swelling.

<u>Poisoning: SAMPLE</u>
(Signs/Symptoms, Allergies, Medications, Past medical history, Last meal, Events)

S - Signs/Symptoms

- **What to Do:** Identify, observe and note any signs and/or symptoms such as nausea, vomiting, confusion, or difficulty breathing.

A - Allergies

- **What to Do:** Check if the person has any known allergies to substances, food, or medications.

M - Medications

- **What to Do:** Gather information about any medications the person is taking.

P - Past Medical History

- **What to Do:** Ask about past medical history and attempt to understand if there are any underlying medical conditions.

L - Last Meal

- **What to Do:** Determine the last meal that they had. This can help understand if food poisoning might be involved.

E - Events

- **What to Do:** Identify and gather details about the events leading up to the symptoms.

<u>Hypothermia: COLD</u>
(Cover, Overexertion, Layers, Dry)

C - Cover

Cover the person with warm blankets.

- **What to Do:** Use blankets, warm clothing, or body heat to warm the person.

O - Overexertion

Avoid overexertion.

- **What to Do:** Keep the person calm and still to prevent further heat loss.

L - Layers

Layer clothing to insulate.

- **What to Do:** Use multiple layers of clothing to trap heat.

D - Dry

Keep the person dry.

- **What to Do:** Remove any wet clothing and replace it with dry, warm items.

<u>Allergic Reactions: EPI</u>
(Epinephrine, Position, Identify)

E - Epinephrine

Administer epinephrine.

- **What to Do:** Use an EpiPen if available (see pg16 for detailed instructions.

P - Position

Position the person properly.

- **What to Do:** Keep them lying down with legs elevated if they feel faint or are in shock.

I - Identify

Identify the allergen.

- **What to Do:** Try to determine what caused the allergic reaction and avoid further exposure.

General First Aid: DRSABCD
(Danger, Response, Send for help, Airway, Breathing, Circulation, Defibrillation)

D - Danger
Check for danger. Ensure the area is safe for you and the victim.

R - Response
Check for a response. Tap and shout to see if the person responds.

S - Send for Help
Call for emergency assistance. Dial 911 or your local emergency number.

A - Airway
Open the airway. Tilt the head back and lift the chin to open the airway.

B - Breathing
Check for breathing. Look, listen, and feel for normal breathing.

C - Circulation
Provide chest compressions. Perform CPR with chest compressions and rescue breaths.

D - Defibrillation
Use a defibrillator if available. Follow the instructions on an automated external defibrillator (AED) if one is available.

Your Call to Action: Be the Difference in an Emergency

Emergencies strike without warning, turning ordinary moments into critical situations where every second counts. The ability to act swiftly and correctly can be the difference between life and death. Throughout this book, we've debunked common myths and misconceptions surrounding emergency first aid, replacing them with clear, actionable steps designed to empower you in those crucial moments.

Knowledge is Power

Understanding the correct procedures for handling medical emergencies is not just about possessing information—it's about being prepared to save lives. Whether it's recognizing the signs of a stroke, correctly administering an EpiPen, or knowing how to stop severe bleeding, your knowledge and actions can profoundly impact the outcome of an emergency.

Facing Fear with Confidence

In emergencies, fear and panic can be paralyzing. This book has equipped you with the tools to face such situations with confidence. By demystifying first aid techniques and providing straightforward, easy-to-follow instructions, we've aimed to make these potentially overwhelming scenarios more manageable. Remember, staying calm and focused is crucial to effectively helping someone in need.

Empathy and Reassurance

Beyond the technical skills, we've emphasized the importance of empathy and communication. Providing reassurance and support to a person in distress is as critical as the medical intervention itself. Your calm and comforting presence can help alleviate fear and anxiety, making the entire experience less traumatic for everyone involved.

A Portable Guide for All

Designed to be a compact, no-nonsense resource, this booklet fits easily into your purse, pocket, or glove compartment. Its purpose is to be readily accessible whenever and wherever you need it. Whether you're at home, at work, or on the road, this guide ensures you're never without the essential knowledge needed to respond to emergencies.

Your Role as a First Responder

Remember, you don't need to be a medical professional to make a difference. As a first responder, your timely and informed actions can stabilize a situation until professional help arrives. This book has provided you with the basics, but continuous learning and practice are key to maintaining and enhancing your skills.

Stay Informed, Stay Prepared

Medical knowledge and guidelines evolve, so staying informed about the latest first aid techniques is crucial.

Consider taking a certified first aid course, attending refresher sessions, and keeping up-to-date with current medical advice. Being prepared means continuously building on the foundation laid by this book.

Final Thoughts

Emergencies are unpredictable, but your ability to respond effectively doesn't have to be. By absorbing the knowledge within these pages, you're taking a significant step towards becoming a capable and confident first responder. Equip yourself with this life-saving wisdom, share it with others, and carry it with you always. You never know when you'll need it, but when the time comes, you'll be ready.

Thank you for taking the time to read this book and for your commitment to being prepared. Together, we can make a difference, one informed action at a time.

Christopher Markus

<u>Disclaimer</u>

The information provided in this book, **Your Pocket Guide to Saving Lives: Debunking Common Myths & Misconceptions and Mastering Emergency First Aid**, is intended for general knowledge and educational purposes only. It is not a substitute for professional medical advice, diagnosis, or treatment. Always seek the advice of your physician or other qualified health provider with any questions you may have regarding a medical condition.

In an emergency, it is crucial to contact emergency services and seek professional medical assistance immediately. The techniques and instructions outlined in this book are meant to provide basic first aid guidance and are not comprehensive medical training.

The author and publisher of this book are not responsible for any adverse effects or consequences resulting from the use of the information provided. The use of this book and the information contained within it is at the reader's own risk.

www.ingramcontent.com/pod-product-compliance
Lightning Source LLC
Chambersburg PA
CBHW050813250726

48653CB00006B/2205